MASSAGE BASICS FOR MASSAGE NERDS

MARIA NATERA

Copyright © 2022 Maria Natera

All rights reserved.

DEDICATION

Whether you are a recent student or a seasoned therapist, you will find value in the wisdom & lessons in this book.

This book might not make you a better massage therapist; however, it can help you look like you know what you are doing! Fake it until you make it.

CONTENTS

INTRODUCTION (1)

1: EACH STATE AND COUNTRY HAS ITS OWN RULES AND REGULATIONS (3)

2: KNOW WHEN TO ETHICALLY REFER YOUR CLIENT TO ANOTHER THERAPIST (4)

3: BE THE THERAPIST THAT LISTENS MORE THAN THEY TALK! (6)

4: BE THE THERAPIST THAT LISTENS TO THE CLIENT'S NEEDS! (8)

5: BE FLEXIBLE (10)

6: MASSAGE FOR THE FULL AMOUNT OF TIME ADVERTISED (11)

7: BE THE THERAPIST THAT LEADS BY EXAMPLE (12)

8: LEAVE YOUR PHONE OUTSIDE THE MASSAGE ROOM! (13)

9: DON'T WAIT UNTIL YOU BURN OUT (14)

10: BE PUNCTUAL (15)

11: BE AWARE THAT THE CLIENTS HAVE DIFFERENT NEEDS ON DIFFERENT DAYS (16)

12: BE PROFESSIONAL AT ALL TIMES (17)

13: LOOK UP ANY HEALTH ISSUES BEFORE YOUR CLIENT SHOWS UP FOR THE APPOINTMENT (19)

CHAPTER 14: TAKE GOOD DOCUMENTATION (20)

15: SET HEALTHY BOUNDARIES WITH YOUR CLIENTS (21)

16: HAVING YOUR TABLE READY AND SET WHEN THE CLIENT COMES IN IS CONDUCIVE TO RELAXATION (23)

17: KEEP YOUR LICENSES CURRENT (24)

18: SCOPE OF PRACTICE (25)

19: ASK CLIENTS FOR FEEDBACK (26)

20: BE CONFIDENT WHEN YOU GIVE A MASSAGE (27)

21: NEVER STOP LEARNING (29)

22: MAKE YOUR CLIENT FEEL LIKE THEY ARE THE MOST IMPORTANT PERSON (30)

23: DON'T COMPARE YOURSELF TO ANOTHER THERAPIST (31)

24: BE FLEXIBLE WHEN THE CLIENT REQUIRES ADJUSTMENTS (32)

25: TAKE PRIDE IN THE SERVICES YOU PROVIDE (33)

26: DON'T HIDE IN THE BATHROOM TO

READ YOUR TEXT
MESSAGES (34)

27: MUSIC CAN
CREATE A RELAXING
ATMOSPHERE (35)

28: WALK YOUR
CLIENT TO THE
MASSAGE ROOM AND
CLOSE THE DOOR
FOR THEM (36)

29: BE AWARE OF
NONVERBAL CUES
(37)

30: BE MINDFUL OF
PEOPLE WITH
ALLERGIES (38)

31: BE OPEN TO
CHANGE (39)

32: IF YOU HAVE A
CLIENT FOR THE
FIRST TIME, EXPLAIN
WHAT YOU MEAN BY
"UNDRESS" (40)

33: IF YOU WANT TO
BUILD UP A
CLIENTELE,
SCHEDULE YOUR
CLIENT'S
APPOINTMENT
BEFORE THEY LEAVE
(41)

34: FOLLOW UP WITH FIRST-TIME CLIENTS IN A DAY OR TWO (42)

35: RELAXATION AND HEALING BEGIN WITH THE NERVOUS SYSTEM (43)

36: KNOW THAT YOU ARE VALUED (46)

37: GIVE YOURSELF PERMISSION TO HAVE FUN AND ENJOY WHAT YOU DO (47)

38: HAVE A SIDE HUSTLE (48)

39: KEEP YOUR MASSAGE ROOM NEAT AND CLEAN (49)

40: KEEP YOUR NAILS TRIMMED AND CLEAN (50)

41: STAY HYDRATED (51)

42: ALWAYS BE READY BEFORE YOUR CLIENT ARRIVES (52)

43: DRESS APPROPRIATELY (53)

44: DON'T BE THE DRIPPY, SMELLY THERAPIST (54)

45: KEEP THE TEMPERATURE COMFORTABLE FOR YOUR CLIENT (55)

46: KEEP A TOOTHBRUSH, MOUTHWASH, MINTS, GUM, OR WHATEVER YOU NEED TO KEEP YOUR BREATH FRESH (56)

47: STAY HOME IF YOU ARE SICK (57)

48: WASH YOUR HANDS BEFORE AND AFTER EVERY MASSAGE (58)

49: SCHEDULE ENOUGH TIME BETWEEN YOUR CLIENTS (59)

CLOSING (60)

ACKNOWLEDGMENTS

I would like to acknowledge my son Chef André Natera for inspiring me to write this book. Without his help, encouragement, and belief in me, this book would not have been possible.

I would also like to give a special thanks to Caryl Barkin. She started and set up my YouTube channel. Her commitment, unconditional love, and support made it possible to have 149,000 subscribers and reach massage therapists around the world.

INTRODUCTION

I've been a massage therapist for 35 years. I graduated from massage school in 1988. I've worked on over twenty-thousand clients and taught hundreds of students since 1995. I graduated from The University of Texas at El Paso (UTEP) Cum Laude with a bachelor's degree in Health Sciences. I started my YouTube channel in 2019 to connect and help massage therapists around the world. When I started my career as a massage therapist, I was an entrepreneur even before the word was popular. I was network marketing even though I didn't know what it meant at the time. I built my career from the bottom up, one massage at a time. I provided professional massage therapy and built my practice by word-of-mouth referrals.

When students graduate from massage school, they are so eager and excited to get into the workforce and start reaping the financial and emotional rewards of the hard work they have just endured. Most of the time it is a difficult transition. Some want to start off with their own business and skip the experience they can gain by putting in the hard work. The reality of giving massages during their internship is different from going to work for a spa, chiropractor, massage establishment, or becoming self-employed. It takes practice and repetition to gain experience before you can be ready to venture out in your own business. I advise students to put in at least a year or two working for someone else so they can gain experience. There is so much that goes into being self-employed. Even though we talk about it in the classroom, it is different in real life.

My goal is to help all students transition into the workforce as easily and as positively as possible. The reality is that after students graduate and receive their certification, only about half of the students take the MBLEx test. The MBLEx is the state-required test for all students to become registered in their state. This test is for USA residents only if this does not apply to you check your country's regulations. Some students fail the first time they take the test and they may get discouraged. It becomes difficult to continue, especially when the pressures of life start getting in the way, and they don't have the support from family, instructors, and peers to help motivate them after the program. Once they receive their certification, it is up to them to follow through with the registration in their State.

I saw a need to help these students transition into the professional world of massage therapy. I wrote this book to help all massage therapists find the motivation, the instruction, and some answers to help them become professional massage therapists. Avoiding the pitfalls that lead to failure.

CHAPTER 1: EACH STATE AND COUNTRY HAS ITS OWN RULES AND REGULATIONS

The licensing board of each state varies in its regulations. It is important for a therapist to stay current with their region's regulations. They should not just familiarize themselves with the regulations but also find out why some massage therapists have complaints filed against them or lose their licenses. This will help prevent those issues from being repeated.

According to Fitch (2015), there are physical boundaries, emotional boundaries, professional boundaries, and social boundaries that all massage therapists need to be familiar with. The most common complaint in my state of Texas is sexual misconduct. Under the Code of Ethics, massage therapists "shall not engage in sexual contact during a session with a client" 16 Tex. Admin. Code S117.92(a). Other common complaints against Texas massage therapists include everything from criminal history, practicing without a license, sanitation issues, ethics, improper techniques, fraud, false advertising, and failure to provide mandatory consultation documentation.

The laws are made by the state government. Rules are made by the regulators to ensure compliance with the law. During the pandemic, some changes were implemented. I remember how many of us were confused as to what was required to do or not do during this time. You do not want to act on misinformation, so it is best to know where you can look it up and stay current. I can't emphasize enough how important it is for you to become familiar with the laws, rules, and regulations of your state and country where you are practicing massage therapy.

CHAPTER 2: KNOW WHEN TO ETHICALLY REFER YOUR CLIENT TO ANOTHER THERAPIST

This has been a question that some therapists might not consider an option. In my years of experience, there have been times that I had to refer a client to another therapist. We are all human and sometimes we have clients that may trigger us. If you are not comfortable with the client for any reason you do not have to keep them as a client. You have the right to terminate services without having to give an explanation.

It's important to know the difference between transference and countertransference. Transference is when the client may transfer their feelings, attitudes & experiences from the past to the present situation. Transference can occur when a client's needs were not met in the past and are now being met by the therapist. This can produce powerful feelings of love and affection or the opposite such as feeling uncomfortable with the therapist.

Countertransference is the reverse. It is from the therapist to the client. They can trigger emotions that are uncomfortable for you. This is not the client's fault; however, you might not be able to be objective in your treatment if you are not comfortable. Being attracted to people is human nature however if this is getting in the way of being professional it cannot continue.

Here are some things to look out for!
- Feeling angry or resentful towards the client.
- Obsessive thinking about the client.

- Physically attracted to the client
- Losing patience with a client for no reason.
- Being impatient with a client that is not progressing with your treatment.
- Boundaries are becoming blurred.

It is important as a professional therapist to have a list of professionals that you can refer to when it is needed. I have a list of doctors, orthopedic surgeons, physical therapists, chiropractors, sports medicine physicians, counselors, nutritionists, and other massage therapists. We must stay within our scope of practice and learn to set boundaries with our clients. Knowing when to refer out makes you a professional therapist.

You can learn more by watching my video on YouTube "Scope of Practice".

CHAPTER 3: BE THE THERAPIST THAT LISTENS MORE THAN THEY TALK!

We are born with two ears and one mouth for a reason. I have had plenty of clients tell me throughout the years that they stopped going to a massage therapist because they would talk throughout the session.

"The therapist was really nice, yet they talked throughout the entire session"

The client was polite and accommodating to the therapist! I quickly took note of this and made a conscious choice to establish a routine where I can catch up with my clients for the first 10 or 15 min. then stay quiet for the remainder of the time. Sometimes clients have a difficult time winding down and they need to talk for a bit. After a few minutes, I change their focus by saying something like "try to listen to the music and take some deep breaths". This helps to remind them that it's time to relax and be quiet. Some people are uncomfortable with being quiet. You can help them by letting them know its ok to be quiet and focus on the music. There is an exception to the previous statements. The geriatrics (elderly) population. Sometimes you may be the only person that they talk and vent to. I make an exception with them because they need that interaction.

Don't spend the session talking about your pets or kids or whatever is important to you. Don't put the client in a position where they're uncomfortable listening to your stories. Clients are nice people, and they're not going to tell you they are not interested. Take care of your talking needs before you enter the massage room.

I have received well over 1,000 massages in my life. I can honestly say that the ones I enjoyed the most are the ones where I was completely relaxed and neither one of us talked.

I have several videos on my YouTube channel where I demonstrate giving a massage without talking. Check out the "No talking with music ASMR full body massage".

CHAPTER 4: BE THE THERAPIST THAT LISTENS TO THE CLIENT'S NEEDS!

This is one of the top complaints that clients have about massage therapists. I especially see this with students. They haven't completely learned all the protocols yet, so it's understandable. It's not about how deep you can go, showing off your new techniques, or practicing what you just learned. It's ok in a classroom setting, however, as a professional you do not do this. Yes, you probably know more about the body than your client; yet your client knows more about their own body. Most importantly they know where it hurts!

Some clients feel frustrated when they tell the therapist that they have pain in a certain area and want it to be worked out thoroughly. The therapist proceeds to give a full body massage and only spends 5 to 10 minutes on that area. Clients feel frustrated, and cheated and are thinking throughout the massage, "when are you getting to the place that really hurts and needs attention?"

One way to approach this is to do some reflective listening before you start the session. You repeat back to the client what they have said so that you can be clear as to what they need. Example: "Would you like for me to focus ½ hour on your back; and are you ok with me skimming over the other areas?" Make sure they understand and agree.

I know a lot of you work for different corporations and you must cover yourself so that there will be no misunderstandings, or complaints afterward. You can document your verbal interaction with the client. Reflective listening is the best way to show your client you are listening, and you get them to agree and take responsibility for the adjustments you are making.

Another complaint that I've heard is, "I told the therapist that it was too much pressure," or, "You can go a little deeper," and the therapist never adjusted the pressure to what the client requested. The client is not going to be reminding you every 5 minutes or every time they see you that they either want more pressure or less pressure. They will give up and eventually find another therapist. That's how a lot of clients ended up coming to me. Listen to your clients' needs!

CHAPTER 5: BE FLEXIBLE

I know we all learned a certain routine in school or learned from the best instructors, yet sometimes we need to expand or adjust for the client. If you have a client that has allergies and gets congested (it should be in the medical history) even if your routine is to start supine, you can change it and start them prone or side-lying. This gives their sinuses a chance to clear up when they end in the supine position. I know it's difficult to change our routine and it throws us off. Eventually, you will have a routine for starting in the supine, prone, or side-lying positions. Just do it, be flexible and your client will appreciate your flexibility and ability to accommodate their needs.

CHAPTER 6: MASSAGE FOR THE FULL AMOUNT OF TIME ADVERTISED

I have heard plenty of complaints about this. Many clients would start coming to me because the therapist didn't give them the full time that was paid for. If you go to a place that advertises a 60-minute massage the client expects that. Clients would complain that they would end up only receiving a 50-minute massage. The therapist would say to them that they deducted 10 minutes for changing. If there was a sign indicating this, then it wasn't visible for the client to easily read. The client will end up either frustrated or ready to find another therapist. In some locations, you may be reported for false advertisement, so always know your local rules and regulations.

CHAPTER 7: BE THE THERAPIST THAT LEADS BY EXAMPLE

It's difficult to give suggestions to your clients about wellbeing, health, and taking care of themselves when you don't do it for yourself. Being a massage therapist is physically, mentally, and sometimes emotionally demanding. Giving massages is very physical yet it's different from you exercising. Sometimes clients with a lot of emotional baggage can be draining too. Setting healthy boundaries with your clients is important so they don't dump on you for an hour and leave you feeling like you got hit by a truck. You have the right to protect your mental and emotional state.

It is a delicate balance to keep physical, mental, and emotional health in check. Take time occasionally to check in on yourself. Remember that your health is your wealth!

CHAPTER 8: LEAVE YOUR PHONE OUTSIDE THE MASSAGE ROOM!

Even though it is not a law that you can't take your phone into the massage room, it is unethical. Most professional massage companies do not allow this. Learn the rules of the place where you work at prior to giving your first massage. One reason is that you never want to be accused of taking pictures of a client. It is also a big "NO" to answer a call while the client is on the table! Trust me, I have heard clients complain about this. I have called other massage therapists that answered my call and asked me if they could call me back because they were with a client. I felt bad for the client on the table. Unless you are part of a secret military mission, please don't answer your phone while working on a client because it tells them that they are not your priority at that moment. They are paying for that session, so you are on their time. Breaking contact with your client to answer a phone call is something you should never do during a session. Even if you use Bluetooth, it is still not proper etiquette.

CHAPTER 9: DON'T WAIT UNTIL YOU BURN OUT

Schedule breaks during the day and throughout the year. The average career span of a massage therapist is only seven years! Usually, it's because they burn out or sustain injuries. It is difficult to maintain this job long-term if you don't take breaks. If you are self-employed make sure you leave time in between your clients to drink water, go to the bathroom, and take some deep breaths. Usually, 30 minutes in between clients is enough. Some places only allow you 15 minutes in between clients. When you work for a company where they schedule one client after another, you will always be exhausted at the end of a day of 7-8 massages.

Take a bath. Schedule regular massages for yourself. Schedule three to four vacations a year, even if they are just weekend getaways to sleep in all day in a hotel! I did this several times. I just needed to unplug from everything and everyone. You can't give the same quality of massage when you're drained as when you're rested.

You can check out my video on YouTube "7 Ways to come back from burnout". When you don't enjoy giving massages anymore it's time to take a break. Take care of yourself, and you will be better prepared to take care of others.

CHAPTER 10: BE PUNCTUAL

I've had massages from plenty of therapists in my 35 years as a practitioner. Students, colleagues, massage therapists in other cities, etc. This therapist was my favorite of all time. We'll call her Chona. She is one of the best therapists I've ever known. I would always get there before she did. Sure, there was always the text or call saying she was running a little late. Rushing in setting up the table and starting on me 15-20 minutes late every time. This is what separates the professional from the unprofessional. I loved her massages yet the frustration of waiting and the rushing to set up made it stressful. I still love Chona and we are good friends; however, I did not schedule more massages with her.

Be ready for your client when they walk in through that door. This will show that you care and are ready to give your undivided attention from the moment they walk in. Most of us don't ever get that from anyone so let your client know they are special. This is how we can change the world one massage at a time.

CHAPTER 11: BE AWARE THAT THE CLIENTS HAVE DIFFERENT NEEDS ON DIFFERENT DAYS

Make sure to take a couple of minutes to ask the client what they need that day. I always ask, "how can I help you today". I give them the option to let me know what they need that day. Even if they are on a specific treatment plan, maybe they had a bad week and can't handle the specific work. They may just need a relaxing Swedish massage. Remember it is not about all the techniques you know even though you think that's what the client needs, that day they may not be up for it. The opposite can be true also. If you have a client that always comes in for a Swedish massage maybe that day, they have low back pain and need you to focus more time on that. Be flexible and willing to adjust for them.

CHAPTER 12: BE PROFESSIONAL AT ALL TIMES

Don't share information about other therapists or family members of your clients. This is a violation of confidentiality. Keep conversations professional and don't open the door to an intimate dialogue. Redirect the conversation if a client is trying to engage you in a conversation that is inappropriate or you're not comfortable with. You can also tell them straight out that the conversation is over, and you will not discuss anything personal. Remember that you are in control of the conversation.

I've had many clients that would complain about their previous massage therapist. Most of the time I knew whom they were talking about, so it made me uncomfortable. Our job is to just listen and acknowledge our clients' feelings. Once I said something out loud after seeing a hematoma (bruise) the size of a grapefruit that the previous therapist had left. It had already been a week since the massage and the bruises were still visible. I was upset to hear that the therapist convinced the client that it was normal and part of the therapy. She had let the therapist know several times that it was hurting, and the therapist still didn't back off. It is not okay for me to put down another therapist or talk about them, yet at that moment I reacted, and my comment was very colorful! Please refrain from saying what you are thinking!

After 35 years of private practice, I usually see other family members. Clients would send their spouses, children, parents, friends, and coworkers. They each shared information with me. This information is always private and confidential. I learned from my mistake. I had a client that came in and shared some exciting news with me. The next time her mom came in I said, "Congratulations on becoming a grandma!" She wasn't supposed to know yet, and I spoiled the surprise! I learned a valuable lesson here. Keep your mouth shut and don't share information with anyone else!

CHAPTER 13: LOOK UP ANY HEALTH ISSUES BEFORE YOUR CLIENT SHOWS UP FOR THE APPOINTMENT

Hopefully, you are the one scheduling the appointment with your client and can get some information prior to their session. I teach students that the massage begins on the phone when the client is scheduling the appointment. I know with technology you can also schedule online, so maybe you can include a question like "Are there any health issues I need to be aware of?". This way you can research before you see the client. Sometimes asking other coworkers can help a lot too because they might have experience working with that situation. For example: maybe your coworkers have worked on a client with a sinus infection, and they tell you that side-lying works better than the prone position. Always check before you start working on the client.

CHAPTER 14: TAKE GOOD DOCUMENTATION

When you see several clients a day every day for weeks it is difficult to remember exactly what you did in the previous massage. S.O.A.P. notes can make the difference between winging it and being professional. I've had clients come in after a month and tell me to do the exact same thing that I did a month ago! If I didn't take good notes, I would not remember what I did or which modality I used the previous month. When you document everything that you do it makes it easier to continue the same treatment. In Texas, documentation is actually required every time you see your client. You may need to provide this documentation for insurance purposes, reimbursements, legal matters (if the client is involved in an accident), and medical doctors. I have a video on "S.O.A.P. notes" that you can follow along at Massage Therapeutics on YouTube.

CHAPTER 15: SET HEALTHY BOUNDARIES WITH YOUR CLIENTS

There are different types of boundaries that need to be considered in a therapist/client relationship. Blurry boundaries may lead down a slippery slope and eventually be crossed. Boundaries can be violated both ways. Either the therapist may take advantage of the client, or the client takes advantage of the therapist. Whether they are professional, emotional, social, or physical boundaries they must be established from the beginning.

Most massage therapists are caring, giving, nice, empathetic, and love to help others. Massage therapists are some of the best people I know! Some clients may take advantage of this. It can be challenging to set boundaries when you are self-employed. When you work for someone else the rules are already established for you. For example, some clients habitually run late or cancel at the last minute. After the third time a client runs late, I let them know that I will be deducting the time from their massage. I understand that unexpected things happen sometimes and it's inevitable, yet when it's a habit for them, it's a problem for me. I only work until the scheduled time.

When I'm faced with a situation like this, I joke with my client and tell them that I could still do more in half the time than most therapists. Humor goes a long way to alleviate tension, and clients appreciate it when you are lighthearted. Because I conduct myself as a businesswoman, clients get the message that their failure to be on time was their loss. I've had clients that were doctors, and they were punctual. If they can do it there is no excuse for anyone else in my opinion.

As another example, Sundays were my only day off, yet I found myself working on Sundays many times. There was always the client who would call Sunday morning and ask me for a massage because they were hurting. I couldn't say no to someone who was hurting! I found myself going in almost every Sunday for a client who waited too long to schedule a massage before they had to work on Monday! I really didn't mind doing this in my early years until I started getting older and needed more days to recover and rest. It was difficult to learn to say no, but my body was telling me I needed to stop working on Sundays.

Some people don't value your time, so you need to make sure *you* value your time. Don't let them take advantage of you because you're nice! Set boundaries from the very beginning because it becomes difficult to set them later. You can become angry and resentful at the client that always cancels at the last minute. If you continually allow this, then you can't be upset with the client because it's something you need to fix, not them. Most of the time the clients that I have now are punctual, considerate, give me a 24-hour cancelation notice, don't come in when they are sick, and give good tips. We are all happy at the end of the day because of the boundaries I set. It's a win-win. This is conditioning at its best - used for good instead of evil.

CHAPTER 16: HAVING YOUR TABLE READY AND SET WHEN THE CLIENT COMES IN IS CONDUCIVE TO RELAXATION

Please call it a table and not a bed. I have heard therapists call it a bed. It is not a bed nor an appropriate name for it. The connotation of bed is not a visual you want your clients to have. Making your table look nice and neat is a must. I personally don't like to see wrinkled sheets on the table. I like to make the sheets look as smooth as possible. You can even run your hand over the top to make it look ironed out.

You can add extra foam or cushion to your table to make it feel softer. Adding arm extensions for the clients who need the extra arm space will make them feel more comfortable. Extra bolsters or pillows are a must, especially for pregnant women or the elderly. Your client will be lying on the table for a good while so making them comfortable is important.

I suggest that you leave your table set up before you leave for the day. It makes your room look professional and ready. Feel free to make changes and change your room around. After 20 years of using white sheets, I decided to change it to prints and colors. I wasn't sure if my clients would like the change because I thought it might not look as professional. I found their response refreshing and fun. They would comment on the prints and colors. I soon figured out which were their favorites so I would use those sheets for their session. That was a nice change for me because I did get tired of the white sheets after so many years. I even have my own favorite se

CHAPTER 17: KEEP YOUR LICENSES CURRENT

TDLR (Texas Department Licensing Regulation) requires that you have your license with a current photo and placed it where it is visible to the clients. This is one of the top five complaints according to TDLR. The massage therapist license needs to be renewed every 2 years before the last day of your birth month. Both the Massage Therapy Instructor license and the Massage Establishment license are good for two years and need to be renewed in the same month you applied for them. The Continuing Education license is also good for two years. This is if you want to be an instructor for CEU classes.

I have all four, so imagine the expense of renewing the licenses, which is one of the things to consider if you want to be self-employed. The expiration date is printed on the license, so it is easy to access if you have them on the wall. Believe it or not, I've known massage therapists that forget to renew their license! It is important to keep your license current and displayed with a picture. Make sure you know the licensing rules for your state or country.

CHAPTER 18: SCOPE OF PRACTICE

Know your scope of practice. As massage therapists, we cannot diagnose or assume anything. Even after doing an assessment, we can't tell our clients they have a herniated disk or a torn rotator cuff. These diagnoses are done by a medical doctor usually after an MRI. When you tell the client they have a rotator cuff tear or anything beyond your scope of practice, you upset the client without evidence. Even if you're sure, it is best to suggest they seek medical treatment if you see anything that is out of the norm. I have a video on YouTube that might help you with "Scope of Practice".

CHAPTER 19: ASK CLIENTS FOR FEEDBACK

I recently asked a client, "What is the one thing that you found difficult with new therapists?". If the client is coming in for a specific treatment, sometimes it's difficult for them to articulate what they need. Help the client figure out what type of massage they need and how to achieve their goal. You may want to explain what their options are. Make it easier on them by asking them questions. Helping them make an educated decision is the best way to help a client. At the same time, you are creating trust between yourself and the client. You let them know that they have the final word.

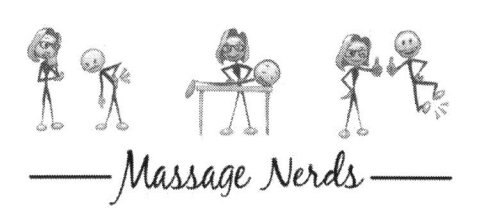

CHAPTER 20: BE CONFIDENT WHEN YOU GIVE A MASSAGE

Pathology can be very intimidating! For a few weeks, all the students hear and learn about is every possible pathology that a client could have. They are scared to hurt the client even if there are no injuries or medical contraindications. Their massage is timid, and it's like they're afraid to touch the client. Not every client is delicate and has a pathology or something wrong with them. The chances are low that you will encounter every pathology in your practice. A good medical history assessment will help you determine if any adjustments will be needed. If you schedule your own appointment, I encourage you to ask your client if there are any issues you need to be aware of before the appointment. That way you have time to research and be prepared before your client comes in.

It is difficult for students with a lack of confidence to transition into a business setting. This is where I say fake it until you make it. Ask the client if there is anything they're aware of that works or doesn't work for them. Remember, they know their body better than you do. They are usually eager to share with you everything that will help them. If you stay within your scope of practice, you will do okay. If you're not doing chiropractic adjustments or forceful ROM (range of motion) or hitting them with a hammer (for those of you that don't know me, I do have a sense of humor), they should be okay. Let them know at the beginning of the session to verbalize if it hurts or becomes uncomfortable. Communication is important when working with clients. The body is not fragile—it can handle a massage. Remember that confidence can be felt through your touch. If you're hesitant the client can feel the hesitation. Fake it till you make it!

CHAPTER 21: NEVER STOP LEARNING

There is always something more to learn. Not that there is anything wrong with doing the same massage routine for years (even though that would be boring for me), yet learning keeps you current and relevant. If it becomes too monotonous, you may lose interest. Here in Texas, we are required to take 12 CE credits as our continuing education. I realize that some classes are expensive; however, there are many ways to learn including trading massages with different people! You will always pick up a new technique from a different therapist.

Both books and social media have excellent resources to learn just about anything. I'd recommend massage therapeutics! After studying massage techniques start delving into the nervous system and the mind. That's when massage therapy becomes very interesting.

There are no excuses for not learning something new. Big or small it doesn't matter. Just continue learning. You create new neurological connections when you learn new things. It helps you improve cognitive functions, improve memory, attention, and mood, and reduce the chance of developing dementia. If you plan a lifelong career in massage, then learning new things is key.

CHAPTER 22: MAKE YOUR CLIENT FEEL LIKE THEY ARE THE MOST IMPORTANT PERSON

I heard someone once say that you are one of two people in the workforce industry. You are either doing the job of three people or are unemployed. Either way, people are tired and stressed. If they are taking the time to schedule an appointment and taking care of themselves, it's our job to deliver. Making them feel cared for and giving them a session of peace and quiet is equivalent to two to three hours of sleep! There are five million touch receptors on our skin! You do make a difference in each client that you see. Helping a client relax and feel better can make a world of difference

CHAPTER 23: DON'T COMPARE YOURSELF TO ANOTHER THERAPIST

Many times, I've heard from colleagues that they can't do eight messages a day. They can't keep up with the young therapist. Every person is unique, and there are many variables that contribute to how many massages you can do a day. I was a single mom with no other support, so I always had something going on with my teenage kids. I was attending university and working towards my bachelor's degree. My parents were still alive, and I was the only child there to help when they needed it. I could never do eight massages a day! On my best days, I did six, max. Once I got into my fifties, I cut back to four. We all need to adjust. Your situation is different from anyone else so don't be hard on yourself. Do what you can do comfortably.

CHAPTER 24: BE FLEXIBLE WHEN THE CLIENT REQUIRES ADJUSTMENTS

I usually start my client supine. Sometimes we need to change our routine. I've had to accommodate clients when they were pregnant and couldn't lay on their stomachs anymore or were too nauseated to lay down. Chair massage comes in handy in some cases. Clients that have had surgery may need to be propped up with a ton of pillows. Clients with COPD need to be at an incline, etc. I've had therapists who weren't taught side-lying and didn't want try it because they didn't feel comfortable working with a client on their side. Don't be afraid to change your routine to accommodate your client. They will be impressed that you can figure out how best to help them, and you will eventually feel comfortable doing a new routine.

CHAPTER 25: TAKE PRIDE IN THE SERVICES YOU PROVIDE

If you say, "Nobody will know if I don't wash the tools or blankets or pillowcases after each client", somebody always knows including you! Massage therapists are some of the cleanest people. We are taught to disinfect and clean our surfaces and laundry. It can be easy to forget the difference between disinfecting, sanitizing, and sterilizing. Disinfecting uses chemicals to kill germs and pathogens. It doesn't necessarily mean cleaning dirty surfaces. It kills germs and lowers the risk of spreading infection. Sanitizing, on the other hand, is removing and lowering the numbers of germs to a safe level set by public health standards. This is what we do as massage therapists.

We sanitize our tools, laundry, and work area. Make sure that you sanitize surface areas! Sterilization is usually used in health care facilities. This is done with steam under pressure, dry heat, hydrogen peroxide, gas plasma, and liquid chemicals. These extreme measures are used in hospitals, laboratories & toxic environments.

Even if you think nobody is watching please sanitize all your tools and blankets or anything else you use during the session. Somebody will always know. Don't cut corners.

CHAPTER 26: DON'T HIDE IN THE BATHROOM TO READ YOUR TEXT MESSAGES

I used to see students leave the classroom to reply to a text. I've done it myself until I caught myself doing it! It's easy for us to excuse ourselves from whatever we are doing to reply to a text. It is very tempting because we live in a society of instant gratification, yet it can wait. Even if you are self-employed, you should not have your phone in the massage room with you. Out of sight out of mind. It can wait. In this world of instant gratification, we need to be reminded that we don't need to reply right away. We need to set boundaries with family and friends also. If we are at work, it's important to let them know to respect our job. If it's not an emergency, it can wait. This is part of conditioning, setting healthy boundaries, and self-discipline.

CHAPTER 27: MUSIC CAN CREATE A RELAXING ATMOSPHERE

The music should be relaxing and conducive to your client's relaxation. The therapist usually plays the type of music that they like to listen to. I can honestly tell you I can't stand Enya. Nothing personal, however, it was the same songs played over & over for years by the same therapist. It's best to have a variety of music readily available. I had a client ask me once to change the music because it sounded like funeral music! I never noticed or thought that, yet it triggered something in her that she didn't like. Ask your clients if they like your music or need it adjusted. The music is about helping your client's relaxation time not about what you personally like.

CHAPTER 28: WALK YOUR CLIENT TO THE MASSAGE ROOM AND CLOSE THE DOOR FOR THEM

I learned this from a colleague. She walks each client to the room and closes the door for them. She mentioned it seemed rude to just let your client walk back by themselves. Even though they know the way to the massage room it is part of giving them your care and attention from the minute they walk in. It's like when your boyfriend would open the car door for you. It just feels good.

CHAPTER 29: BE AWARE OF NONVERBAL CUES

I tell students to learn to listen with their hands, especially when the client is in the prone position because you can't see their facial expressions. If you are paying attention, the body will give you cues. You may be talking with the client; however, if it hurts or feels uncomfortable the nervous system will let you know. They may flinch, move, twitch or jump. There are some obvious clues that you will pick up on. Some are not so obvious, so you need to train your hands to feel - like feeling for different temperatures on the body. If you feel warmth or heat, it could be swelling or an infection, or even a blood clot. If it feels cool or cold to the touch it may be ischemic tissue. Sometimes when you are distracted you may not pay attention to these subtle differences; however, with experience, you will learn to be discerning.

Clients don't always let you know what they're feeling especially if they're in deep relaxation. Sometimes they are not aware of a sensitive area until you touch it. A latent trigger point is when the client doesn't know there is any pain in a certain spot until you touch it. It's like you wake up the tissue, so pay attention to the latent trigger points. Active trigger points, on the other hand, are the ones that the client feels, and they may let you know exactly where it is. Working on both latent and active trigger points is important.

CHAPTER 30: BE MINDFUL OF PEOPLE WITH ALLERGIES

Do you suffer from allergies? Allergy questions should be part of the medical history form, so you know if you need to accommodate someone with allergies. I would schedule my clients with allergies on the same day so I could make sure not to have any smells that would bother them. Don't wear scented lotions, potions, or perfumes around them. You can ask your clients what triggers their allergies. They are usually willing to share with you what works for them. They may bring their own oil or lotion that they prefer. Make sure you ask before you start working on them.

CHAPTER 31: BE OPEN TO CHANGE

I've heard therapists say, "This is the way I've always done it." Be open to learning something new. You never know who can teach you something valuable that you can incorporate into your life. I have taught CE classes, and I see the eagerness of the therapist wanting to learn new things. Whether you're a recent graduate or a seasoned therapist, you never stop learning. It is imperative for our personal growth to continue learning. When you bring fresh ideas and new techniques to your clients, they appreciate the fact that you are learning new things to help them. I found my clients very eager to let me try new techniques on them. Always ask their permission before you try something new.

CHAPTER 32: IF YOU HAVE A CLIENT FOR THE FIRST TIME, EXPLAIN WHAT YOU MEAN BY "UNDRESS"

I've had male clients and females too, ask me what "undress" means? The therapist says something like "I'm going to step out so you can undress". That's it! I had a male client tell me he didn't know what to do. Do I take my underwear off or do I leave them on? He felt uncomfortable the whole time not knowing what he should have done. Please remember that not everyone knows what you expect. I would just add another sentence like "you can leave your underwear on or off - whatever makes you comfortable".

If you have a client who needs work on the deep hip rotators and gluteal muscles, you can explain why it would be beneficial to remove their underwear. I reassure the client that they will be draped the entire time, and I will only work on the muscles that need it. I undrape the side of the glutes that I'm working on. Never show the butt crack line or bring the drape all the way down. You can tuck it in at the waist level on the opposite side of the table and by the trochanter of the femur on the side that you are working on. Never go near genital areas to tuck in the sheet. It's important to make the client feel comfortable and safe from the beginning of the session so explain what you mean.

CHAPTER 33: IF YOU WANT TO BUILD UP A CLIENTELE, SCHEDULE YOUR CLIENT'S APPOINTMENT BEFORE THEY LEAVE

Don't say, "Give me a call when you need to come back," because even if they tell you, "I'll give you a call," they usually don't. People are busy, and they forget or postpone longer than they mean to. It's best to schedule them right then and there. I usually schedule my clients at the same time on the same day so they can remember it more easily They will think, "Today is Wednesday; I have my massage. It will help me make it through the week!" This is conditioning the client, and it is one of the ways I built my clientele.

I have found that Friday evenings were not a good day to schedule clients. Sometimes they just wanted to go home, or something would come up, so they needed to reschedule. I started not scheduling on Friday evenings for this reason. It was the day that I had the most cancelations. Get your client in the habit of scheduling. their appointments before they leave When you are working on a treatment plan with a client, it is best if they schedule each week for three weeks in a row. I have found this works well for caring for injuries. If you wait too long in between massages, it is like starting over again. Clients will see better results when they come in regularly

CHAPTER 34: FOLLOW UP WITH FIRST-TIME CLIENTS IN A DAY OR TWO

It's really a good idea for you to check on your clients after they've had a massage. It will let you know how they did with the pressure you applied. I ask them if they were sore, and if so, how long it lasted. If the soreness lasted more than 48 hours that tells you too much pressure was used. There should not be any bruises either. Asking them how they felt and being open to their feedback will help you adjust their treatment plan. As I mentioned earlier, if you tell your client, "Give me a call and let me know how you felt," they usually don't call you, especially if they don't know what you're looking for. It is best if you call them and ask them specific questions.

There were times when I used too much pressure unwillingly. It is difficult to know how much pressure to use on a first-time client, especially if they tell you to go as deep as you can. It is up to us to learn about their body and listen to their non-verbal cues. If they were sore for longer than 48 hours, I had an opportunity to save face and explain to them that the massage was too deep and next time I would adjust. When you take the time to explain, they appreciate it and learn to trust you. Massage is about the client feeling safe and trusting the therapist

CHAPTER 35: RELAXATION AND HEALING BEGIN WITH THE NERVOUS SYSTEM

I can't emphasize this enough! I remember when I was in massage school, we were taught the nervous system in a couple of hours. It has taken me a lifetime to learn more about how important the nervous system is and the psychology of how the body keeps the score of traumas, whether from an accident or emotional trauma. It's fascinating. I suggest you delve into the depths of the connection between the body and the mind. I recommend *The Body Keeps the Score: Brain, Mind, and Body in the Healing of Trauma* by Bessel Van Der Kolk M.D. It is a great book to start with if you want to learn more about the mind-body connection.

I had a client who had been in a car accident when she was a teenager. She injured her rotator cuff and had surgery. She was now in her forties and ended up on my table because her husband bought her a gift certificate for her birthday. Coming in for a massage was not her idea. I was pleasantly surprised that she continued to come in for two years. The trauma was more than physical because the physical injury had healed 20 years prior, yet she was extremely guarded and sensitive to my touch. She would jump and sometimes scream if I went near that area. I worked on her body except for the rotator cuff muscles for over a year.

It really did take her two years to trust and feel comfortable letting me touch it. I don't think she has worked on the emotional trauma this caused her, however, eventually she trusted me enough to let me massage her shoulder. I just went over it very lightly until her nerve receptors got used to my touch. I would back off if was too much for her—I never forced it. When you are dealing with injuries, whether physical or emotional, you must respect the body. Listen with your hands, and the client's body will lead the way.

Another incident that marked my experience as a massage therapist, happened in my early career. She came in because she too had a shoulder injury. She was extremely quiet and withdrawn. She was the opposite of my first example. She wanted me to work on the shoulder because it had been painful for years, and she was ready to heal. I dedicated the whole hour to working only the muscles related to that shoulder. My modality was neuromuscular, so I addressed everything I knew to do at that time.

During her third session with me, she began to cry uncontrollably. I didn't know what to do because I was a new therapist, only five years in. I had never had anyone cry while on the table before. She sat up, and I brought her tissues and a drink of water. She proceeded to tell me that she had been sexually assaulted nine years prior and her assailant had put her in an arm lock to hold her in place. She had never told anyone, and her shoulder had been damaged ever since. I referred her to a female psychologist who was able to help her work through that traumatic life-changing experience. I never saw her again after that. She did call me to tell me that I had worked out whatever pain she had. It was her emotional release that healed her. She was ready to be healed and wanted me to work on it, unlike the previous client who came in because her husband bought her a gift certificate.

Two different cases, two different reactions, neither were right nor wrong. This is an example of the mind-body connection and how the body can heal itself when it is ready. All we need to do is respect where they are at and do what they allow us to work on. I like to teach that the miracle is the body healing itself. We may assist the body in healing, yet it is the body doing the healing. This keeps our ego in check.

CHAPTER 36: KNOW THAT YOU ARE VALUED

I know sometimes we don't feel confident that we know enough, or imposter syndrome makes us doubt ourselves. Just remember that your client is coming to you because they feel comfortable with you. Your intention to help, soothe, heal, or give what your client needs is enough. They appreciate you! They don't care if you don't know all the names of the muscles or bones or whatever you think you don't know. It really is the intent that you have that transcends anything else.

This world needs more kindness. Massage therapists are some of the best people in the world! I see that now with my YouTube channel with followers from all over the world. We are basically the same whether you live in India, Taiwan, Philippines, Iran, Japan, Mexico, Colombia, Italy, Greece, Spain, etc. The comments from each therapist are basically the same. I can tell they are caring, patient, kind, giving, and amazing. We just want to help others. If you have a clientele, you can be assured that they do like and appreciate you! Don't let imposter syndrome get the best of you! You are enough!

CHAPTER 37: GIVE YOURSELF PERMISSION TO HAVE FUN AND ENJOY WHAT YOU DO

I have been a massage therapist for 35 years now. I am very passionate about doing what I do. I have reinvented myself several times. I like to make my clients and students laugh. This world already has too much stress and pain. Laughter is healing. You must recharge and allow yourself to have hobbies or just watch Netflix all day occasionally. Have fun in whatever you do. Life is short. I wish someone had told me years ago that it always works out in the end. I would not have stressed as much. I can say that teaching is so much fun for me. It's like a hobby because I don't see it as a job. The students are the best. They are passionate, fun, full of life, and eager to learn. Have fun at whatever you do.

CHAPTER 38: HAVE A SIDE HUSTLE

I lived month to month for many years. Unfortunately, you don't get rich from being a massage therapist because you can only work so many massages a day and for so many days. Throughout the years I did several things to supplement my income. I've done everything from making Christmas baskets to selling merchandise to pet sitting and house sitting. I have sold candles, oils, massage creams, CBD products, and more. I usually had a side hustle that brought in extra money.

I have been an instructor for a few schools since 1995. This helped to supplement my income. Even though I had my degree I never wanted to stop teaching or being a massage therapist. I didn't start my YouTube channel until the spring of 2019. Now I have 3 jobs, and I'm publishing this book while still writing another book. The point I am trying to make is that it can be difficult to make ends meet as a massage therapist. My suggestion is that you investigate having a way to make other income. Many self-employed massage therapists have no retirement, no 401K, and no medical insurance, so it is challenging. Our work is about wanting to help others. Don't limit yourself to your potential to supplement your income as a massage therapist. There are many ways to make more money in the field, other than just depending on the physical work of giving massages.

CHAPTER 39: KEEP YOUR MASSAGE ROOM NEAT AND CLEAN

There's nothing worse than walking into a room that is cluttered and messy or that has walls filled with certificates and other paperwork. This is where less is best. You want to create an atmosphere that is conducive to relaxation. I've seen massage rooms with wall-to-wall certifications, yet the therapist wasn't any better than someone that had only one displayed. I used to trade massages with a therapist that had her walls & ceiling covered with vines. Literally had trellises with artificial vines, rainbows & butterflies. It Looked like a jungle in there. I was expecting a monkey to jump out at me!

When I was getting my certification to become an elementary teacher, we learned that overcrowded walls are overstimulating. We are already bombarded every day with noise pollution and sensory overload, so create an atmosphere that is inviting, clean, and Zen. Take pride in your room. Making changes is good if you remember to keep it simple, neat, and clean. If you get bored being in the same room for years, change it up every few months. Paint the walls to give them a fresh look. Most of us know we should keep our room tidy and clean. Remember Chona? She would pile up the dirty sheets in one corner until the end of the day! TDLR (Texas Department of Licensing Regulation) requires us to keep dirty laundry in a closed container preferably in a closet or another room.

CHAPTER 40: KEEP YOUR NAILS TRIMMED AND CLEAN

Make it a routine to trim and file your nails on the same day of the week. This makes it easy to remember and get it done. Make sure you file down the sharp edges after you trim them. Some therapists just cut them and don't file them. Sometimes you can feel the sharp edges when you massage, so make sure you cut and file. I have done this every Monday of my career, and there are still times when my nails are a little scratchy or get hang nails during the winter. I suggest a paraffin wax dip or putting lotions on your hands before you go to bed.

I recently traded massages with a therapist who had long nails. I knew the minute I saw her nails that she would not be able to give a specific massage. It was not the best massage nor the worst one, yet I won't trade with her again. I understand some therapists have other jobs and do massage therapy on the side, so keeping their nails trimmed is not always a priority. However, it is unsanitary to have long nails while you massage.

Brushing under your nails is a good, sanitary practice too. I recommend you have a nail clipper, nail brush, and file at work. This way you can be ready every Monday with trimmed smooth nails.

CHAPTER 41: STAY HYDRATED

Drink water in between your clients not during the session. It is best to drink 3-4 ounces in between your clients rather than 12 ounces at once. This will keep you hydrated throughout the day and prevent you from having to take time during a session to use the bathroom. I know that sometimes we just can't hold it, and we need to excuse ourselves to use the bathroom. It happens sometimes. However, when it becomes a habit that you excuse yourself regularly, that's when it becomes a problem that it doesn't sit well with clients. It's also not a good idea to break contact with your client to sip water during the sessions.

I was confused for many years as to how much water I should drink for my size. Here is a formula that I learned in my nutrition class. Take your body weight and divide it by two. That is the number of ounces of water you need to drink a day for your body size. If you weigh 200 lbs., then you would need to drink 100 ounces of water which equals 12.5 glasses of 8 oz. each. I weigh 115 lbs. so that is equal to 57.5 ounces a day. I need to drink 7.5 glasses of water at 8 ounces each glass. This is a big difference between a petite person and a larger person. To say that everyone should drink the same amount of water doesn't make sense to me (I remember when it was a gallon a day for everyone). You do have to consider if you are exercising or perspiring profusely that you must increase and adjust your water intake. It is best to sip water throughout the day than tax your kidneys by drinking too much at once.

CHAPTER 42: ALWAYS BE READY BEFORE YOUR CLIENT ARRIVES

Whether you are self-employed or work for a private industry it's important to be ready. You want to set the tone from the beginning that you will give your client your undivided attention from the minute they walk in. You have the responsibility to set a tone that is conducive to relaxation. Plenty of times clients come in after work, and they are stressed and tired. The last thing they need is to be frustrated because you're not ready, running late, or stressed yourself. I've had clients tell me that the minute they drive up to my clinic they start relaxing. This is called conditioning!

CHAPTER 43: DRESS APPROPRIATELY

If you work for a chiropractor, PT, or private industry you probably have a dress code. If you are self-employed remember that you set the tone of the clientele that you will attract. I started wearing scrubs because it makes me look professional, and I am taken more seriously—especially if I want to work with professionals like doctors, lawyers, dentists, or anyone else in a professional setting. If you choose not to wear a uniform, remember to dress professionally, not provocatively. Shirts should have sleeves so that armpits are covered. Cleavage should not be shown. If you wear shorts, they should not be too short. Capri pants are ideal. When you play the part, you will become the part!

CHAPTER 44: DON'T BE THE DRIPPY, SMELLY THERAPIST

This complaint is more common than you think. Some massage therapists perspire profusely, I have seen it many times in the classroom. You can do different things to minimize discomfort and avoid embarrassment. I have my students wear a headband or bandana. A wrist band works to wipe off the excess perspiration from your face before it drips on the client!

And please wear deodorant. I've had students throughout the years who don't wear deodorant for many reasons. They are usually the holistic naturals that don't want to use antiperspirants. There are deodorants without aluminum and salt stones that help neutralize body odor. These students were the nicest ones, yet nobody wanted to trade massages with them because they smelled bad! This is a sure way to keep a client from returning. They won't tell you because most people will not say, "You smell." Trust me; I know. I've dealt with clients coming to me because they couldn't tell the therapist themselves. They just won't return. Clients don't want to be put in an uncomfortable situation and give the therapist negative feedback.

CHAPTER 45: KEEP THE TEMPERATURE COMFORTABLE FOR YOUR CLIENT

I can honestly tell you that this is a big challenge for me. I get very hot easily which can make work unbearable. However, I need to adjust to keep my clients happy. During the winter I have a heated pad that keeps the table warm. They love it when they get under the covers. During the summer I may have an extra fan going or frozen bottled water in my scrubs pocket to keep me cool. I recently discovered a neckband that can be dipped in ice water to keep cool. Giving massages can be a workout! I want to be comfortable too so that I can give my client the best of myself.

CHAPTER 46: KEEP A TOOTHBRUSH, MOUTHWASH, MINTS, GUM, OR WHATEVER YOU NEED TO KEEP YOUR BREATH FRESH

If you had garlic the night before, you could still smell it on your breath the next day. All of us must eat lunch during the work day, so make sure you brush your teeth after lunch before you start working on your clients. I'm obsessed with gum, which is not always a good idea, yet it worked for me. Mints work too; however, they dissolve after 10 minutes, and a breath of fire will seep through.

Watch what you eat before you work on clients. It's best not to have a lot of carbohydrates or sugary foods because that will only make you tired and sleepy. Eat healthy snacks in between clients if you need some energy. My go-to snack is always a banana! Packed with nutrients and easy to peel and eat. Sliced oranges and nuts are a great snack too. Snacks that won't smell, are easy to open, and are nutritious are the best.

CHAPTER 47: STAY HOME IF YOU ARE SICK

It is better to reschedule a client than take the chance of spreading something. I think the pandemic has made this more important than ever. Teach your clients why it's important not to come in when they are sick. I would think it is obvious to everyone, yet some people may not be aware of the reasons for this necessity. We are in proximity to our clients in an enclosed room. If you feel sick, you won't be able to give your client the same massage as when you are well. The same applies to the client. When you are working on the body, it may speed up circulation and the lymphatic system. We do work on these systems when we give a massage. Clients usually end up feeling worse the next day, so it is not recommended to receive or give a massage if you are sick.

The common cold is the most contagious illness in schools, and it can easily be spread to other people. I know some people have mild symptoms, yet some people feel bad and have a fever even with just a cold. Please be considerate of others, especially clients with compromised immune systems. It's our ethical duty to protect vulnerable clients with low immune systems. I have turned clients away that came in while they were sick because they didn't think much of it. I needed to protect myself from catching anything to protect my elderly, clients with cancer. I never want to expose them to anything that can jeopardize their health.

CHAPTER 48: WASH YOUR HANDS BEFORE AND AFTER EVERY MASSAGE

I know this sounds like common sense because you are taught this in school. However, this is also a complaint that I have heard about before. I have received questions from some of my followers on YouTube that really surprised me. Some cultures seem to believe that washing your hands after a massage may cause arthritis, especially if you wash them in cold water. Arthritis is caused by the inflammation of the joints. It is usually associated with age and other variables. There is no research that shows that washing your hands after a massage causes arthritis, whether it is with cold or hot water. Just wash your hands. I wash my hands and arm up to my elbows after every massage. I use elbows and forearms so for me it is important to scrub like the doctors do all the way to my elbows. No, I don't sing the happy birthday song. I just count to thirty because that's how long it takes me to wash up to my elbows.

CHAPTER 49: SCHEDULE ENOUGH TIME BETWEEN YOUR CLIENTS

I usually give myself thirty minutes in between clients. That was enough time for me to change the sheets, drink water, and go to the bathroom. Some therapists might need half an hour to accomplish that. They may need to make phone calls, eat a snack, or take care of something else. Do what works for you unless you work for an industry that only allows you a certain time in between your clients. Then it's up to you to prioritize what's important, though I know we've learned to multitask.

LET'S CHANGE THE WORLD ONE MASSAGE AT A TIME!

CLOSING

If you have read this far, I would like to thank you. Thank you to all the thousands of clients and hundreds of students, followers, supporters, colleagues, friends, and family. It is not I who has helped you, it is you who have motivated me every morning to get up and give my best. You have motivated me to learn that new technique or muscle action, and learn how to teach better so that students had fun and learned at the same time. I started having the students paint the muscles on the body 25 years ago. I have students that have made me so proud by seeing how they have succeeded and are far better than I ever was.

The comments on my YouTube from followers from all over the world are overwhelmingly kind and generous. I thank my colleagues for brainstorming about different situations with clients and the many times I needed to vent. They helped with ideas for my videos and different approaches to teaching. I thank my friends who had my back when I was physically and mentally exhausted and ready to quit. I thank my family for putting up with me. I am humbled by the support and the love people have shown me. I do believe we can change the world one massage at a time.

Create a great day.
Maria

ABOUT THE AUTHOR

Maria N. Natera graduated from massage school in 1988 and has had a successful private practice for 35 years. She started teaching at El Paso Community College massage therapy program in 1995. She left a few years later to pursue her own bachelor's degree in Health Sciences from the University of Texas at El Paso. She also taught for the Austin School of massage and is now back teaching at EPCC, fulfilling her passion to help others live a healthy life. She started her YouTube channel in February of 2019 and leads an entrepreneur lifestyle as an instructor, social media presence, private practice, and author.

Printed in Great Britain
by Amazon